Herbal Medicine Guide for Beginners

All you need to know about how to use Medicinal Herbs and Natural Remedies for Self Healing

The information in the following pages is broadly considered to be truthful and accurate account of facts, and as such any inattention, use or misuse of the information in question by the reader will render any resulting actions solely under their purview. There are no scenarios in which the publisher or the original author of this work can be in any fashion deemed liable for any hardship or damages that may befall them after undertaking information described herein.

Additionally, the information in the following pages is intended only for informational purposes and should thus be thought of as universal. As befitting its nature, it is presented without assurance regarding its prolonged validity or interim quality. Trademarks that are mentioned are done without written consent and can in no way be considered an endorsement from the trademark holder.

Table of Contents

Introduction

Congratulations on downloading Herbal Medicine Guide for Beginners and thank you for doing so.

The following chapters will discuss a basic overview of the history of medicinal herbs, from the first man to when herbal medicines became a trading commodity of the world. You will learn the definitions for all of the forms that medicinal herbs can take, what is in the label, and what to look for on the shelf.

There are three chapters providing you with choices of medicinal herbs to treat ailments physically, mentally, and emotionally. Also, we will bring you back to where early man started, being in-charge of your health through the creation of your own medicinal herb garden.

All of the information contained within is practical advice, easy to follow, and designed for your well-being. We encourage you to make medicinal herbs part of your medicine chest and hopefully, part of your everyday health regime. Safer than pharmaceutical options for many of the more common afflictions, medicinal herbs may be the best investment you can make for your future. This guide will lead you into a better quality of life through a deeper appreciation for the world of medicinal herbs.

There are plenty of books on this subject on the market, thanks again for choosing this one! Every effort was made to ensure it is full of as much useful information as possible, please enjoy!

Chapter 1:
A Brief History of Medicinal Plants & Herbs

The English Oxford defines a medicinal plant: *(of a substance or plant) having healing properties.*

Today, a medicinal plant is recognized as one which is used for the maintenance of health and/or to be taken to alleviate a specific ailment. This recognition takes place both in modern and traditional forms of medicine. It was conservatively estimated that there are over 17,810 species of plants which have a use for medicinal purposes out of the 30,000 plants documented for possessing a use of any kind. (The Royal Botanic Gardens, Kew, 2016)

Plants, many of which we recognize today as culinary herbs and spices, have been considered since pre-historic times as containing medicinal value. Humans originated with a close connection to their immediate environment, using what was available to them for food and medicine. Flowering plants are the original source of most medicines. These tended to grow near human settlements, such as chickweed, yarrow, dandelion, and nettles. The trial and error approach was taken when these early 'scientists' applied these sources as potential plants to meet their needs. The knowledge gained was transferred from each generation through oral and written traditions, depending on the culture involved. This knowledge has been gradually becoming more complete as civilizations formed and the sharing of knowledge occurs.

Not only do humans use their environment as a source of medicine, animals including primates, sheep, and monarch butterflies, also consume certain medicinal plants when ill.

The earliest evidence known for the use of plants as medicine comes from prehistoric burial sites. Dating back to the Paleolithic period, a 60,000-year-old Neanderthal site in Iraq contained quantities of pollen from eight plant species, seven of which we use today as remedies.

The earliest written evidence comes from clay tablets dating back to the Sumerian civilization. Recorded on them are hundreds of plants, including opium, used for their medicinal values. Papyrus scrolls from ancient Egypt offer details of eight hundred and fifty plant-based medicines. The source of pharmacopeias, *De materia medica*, documented more than 1,000 medicine recipes based on over six hundred different plant sources. This sourcebook was used for over 1,500 years as a reliable resource for medicinal products.

Before 500 B.C., belief systems at that time ascribed both magical and healing properties to plants. Beginning with the age of Hippocrates, after 500 B.C., physical illness was seen as part of the natural human condition and plants began to lose their mythical properties.

Before the 16th century, there are three widely recognized ancient medicinal systems namely the Chinese medicine, European, and Ayurvedic (Indian). All three are based on very different approaches to the human body but all are in agreement with one essential concept. If the body is out of balance, then illness will result. The restoration of balance is required for good health to be present. One should work with nature and the body's own healing capacity complemented by healing herbs to restore balance.

As part of this shared belief system, all three medical practices held, at their core, a belief that each human contains a primal (vital) energy source. This source sustains the health and life and each individual has it to varying degrees. The Chinese defined this source as "qi" and the Ayurvedic's referred to it as "prana". Westerners referred to it simply as the "vital force".

When world trade exploded in the 14th century, the exchange of remedies and herbs between Muslims, the Chinese, Indians, and Europeans increased. Europeans now add access to new herbs and their healing properties, such as ginger, cinnamon, and cardamom. The Far East was introduced to sage and its potential health benefits at the same time.

Unfortunately, European medicine was not able to treat the many plagues and epidemics that swept through the continent during the 12th and 18th centuries. One common modern day interpretation of the Black plague nursery rhyme *Ring around the Rosie* is that people at the time believed you contracted the disease from breathing 'bad air'. So carrying a posy (sachet) of flowers in your pocket would sweeten the air around you, thus ensuring the carrier would not breathe in any disease.

Herbs brought to Europe from Central and South America, thanks to the Spanish and Portuguese explorers, were potent remedies for successfully treating smallpox, syphilis, and malaria. There followed a surge in popularity for homeopathy and herbal medicines.

In the 19th century, the modern medicine took over, dismissing all previously held concepts of herbal medicine as ignorance and superstition. This was the dawning of the age of western medicine and more traditional practices were overshadowed all over the world.

When the British moved in to colonize India, they declare that the practice of Ayurveda was inferior to western medicine and subsequently tried to squash and replace this traditional form.

China, through the maintenance of closing themselves off the Western world, was more successful at maintaining their traditional medical practices. In many western countries, it became illegal to practice herbal medicine without receiving an official qualification.

People continue to access the healing powers of many plants and herbs, visiting naturopaths, shamans, homeopaths, herbologists, etc. In 1991, the World Health Organization (WHO) formulated a policy on the use of traditional medicines. They have since then published guidelines on the more widely used ones. WHO has estimated, due to a lack of reliable data, up to 80% of our current world population relies on traditional medicine, with approximately two billion of these mainly reliant on medicinal plants. One reason for this is the affordability of plant-based medicines making them more accessible to many people.

In developed countries, there is an increase in the use of plant-sourced medicines which include health care or herbal care products. The benefits from these sources are not always scientifically known as there has been no means of testing the pharmaceutical benefits of each dosage. Since the medicinal value of each plant is dependent on many variables like the soil, sun, a strain of plant, and time of harvesting, it is difficult to assess the benefits and toxicity of these remedies. Although many of these herbal remedies have been in use since early man, there is still very little knowledge of the pharmacological base for their status as a medicinal plant.

Current drug research does make use of ethnobotany to look for active medicinal substances in plants. This research has produced the discovery of hundreds of compounds which are all useful to the medical industry. The most common ones we know of are aspirin (willow bark), quinine, (Remijia bark or Cinchona bark), opium (dried latex from the opium poppy), and digoxin (foxglove flower).

Over a quarter of modern drugs prescribed to patients are sourced from medicinal plants and are rigorously tested prior to use. In some non-industrialized countries, medicinal plants can make up the majority of treatments without the same scientific research. Although there is still little regulation, WHO still does coordinate a network for the safe and practical use of such plants.

Today, there is an annually global export market value of several hundred billion USD in 2017. This market is made up of up to 70,000 plants with anticipated medicinal values. Given that there is little regulation worldwide in the market, medicinal plants face the threat of over-collection to meet demands. Furthermore, climate change and on-going habitat destruction are affecting the viability of these potent medicinal sources. By actively engaging in a deeper awareness of traditional medical knowledge, we can play a key role in a sustained exploitation of these natural resources.

In almost every culture in the world, plants are used as a medical resource. In industrialized nations, the efficacy, safety, and quality of these plants (herbal drugs) have very recently become a key issue. Through the standardization and evaluation of the active plant-derived medical compounds, medicinal plants can assist as an emerging boon to our current healthcare system. Herbal drugs could be the stimulus for future cures of many human diseases. Collaboration with different cultures on their medicinal plant practices is required for the creation of historically accurate accounts for the benefit of the people all over the world.

Beyond their medicinal value, medicinal plants have the potential to increase the quality of life through socio-economic benefits. There is the financial benefit to those who cultivate them for sale, in addition to job opportunities, income via taxation, and a healthier labor force worldwide. The market should be encouraged and further developed through improved practices in the processing and distribution, further scientific research into their medicinal value, and improved financing for those trying to cultivate them.

In the United States most herb product manufacturers already have their products sourced through domestic and foreign markets. The medicinal herb manufacturing industry has been in a steady growth for a number of years and it has matured. Note the number of products readily available in grocery stores, pharmacies, even dollar stores. Probably the best method of purchasing choice organically grown medicinal herb products is by buying products made from from small local manufacturers. Because these companies do not buy in the amounts internationals do they will be the ones purchasing from the local farmer closest to them. By supporting local business you are encouraging diversity and sustainability in the medicinal herb products market.

Chapter 2:
What to Look For In Your Modern Day Medicinal Herbs and Where to Find Them

In this chapter, we will use herb and plant interchangeably with the understanding that an herb is the whole or part of a whole plant which, for the definition of this Guide, is used for its medicinal properties.

Herbal products are defined as being formulated from plants to treat diseases and maintain health. These can come in the form of gels, lotions, salves, ointments, and creams which can be applied directly to your skin. Some products are water soluble and are used in the bath.

There are also essences where the volatile oil of the herb is extracted through a steam distillation. The resulting oil can then be added to your bath, inhaled as a scent, or rubbed on the skin. Some oil like that of oregano is even ingested internally defining this one as a supplement rather than a product.

Poultices and plasters, which involve a soft collection of plant material, are laid on the afflicted body part to relieve the swelling and inflammation. This mass is typically held in place with a cloth.

Herbal supplements are products made from plants and designed only for internal use. These can contain parts of or the whole plant itself. Herbal supplements are sold as pills, tablets, powders, extracts, tinctures, teas, dried, and fresh cuttings of the plant itself.

Pills are used as a general term to define either a capsule or a tablet. They are round and oval, whereas a tablet is flat and circular.

A tablet, which is made up of compressed powder in a solid form, is designed to be cut into two parts.

Capsules contain either a powder or a jelly in a dissolvable gel container. The contents of the capsules are dissolved into the bloodstream immediately.

Teas, also known as infusions, are created by soaking the fresh or dried herbs in hot water and letting them seep. These can then be drunk cold or hot.

A decoction is created by simmering the bark, roots, or berries in hot water for long periods of time. These can also be consumed hot or cold.

Tinctures are created through the soaking of an herb in an alcohol and water solution. This process concentrates and preserves the active ingredients in the herb. Tinctures can vary in their strength and are expressed through a ratio of the weight of the dried herb to the volume of the finished product. Extracts involve soaking the plant in a solvent which removes certain types of chemicals. The resulting liquid can be used as is or evaporated to create a dry powder for use in tablets or capsules.

In 1994, in the United States, the Dietary Supplement Health and Education Act became law. As defined by Congress, a supplement for safe use is one which:

- is used with the intention of supplementing the diet.

- contains one or more of the following as ingredients – herbs, botanicals, amino acids, vitamins, minerals, and other substances,

- the intention is to ingest this orally as a liquid, pill, tablet, capsule, tea, or tincture,

- is clearly and accurately labeled on the front of the bottle as a supplement.

Herbal supplements can range in effect from a mild action with very subtle effects noted over a long period of time to very potent results. Many of the liquid supplements have varying strengths, dependent on if it is a tea, a tincture, or even an extract. A difference in how the supplement is prepared and the concentration of the chemical recovered from the plant can affect the outcome of how it is used. For example, peppermint tea is a fairly mild digestive aid but peppermint oil is very concentrated and can be toxic if not taken correctly. It is important to read the labeling on the supplement or, if you are using the whole herb, consult with a professional for an accurate dosage.

Since the FDA does not consider herbal supplements as drugs (they are classified as food under the Act), they are not subject to the same testing and regulatory standards as drugs. On the labels, the supplements list how the herbs can influence different physical responses but they are not allowed to say they can treat specific conditions.

Determining a manufacturer's claims of quality can depend on hearsay, a doctor's opinion, or even the label itself. Since 2007, there has been something called the Good Manufacturing Process for dietary supplements. These are a list of requirements and expectations which manufacturers have to adhere to for the identification, concentration, purity, and quality of their product. This is in an attempt to prevent the wrongful inclusion of contaminated ingredients, an imbalance of ingredients, and the improper labeling of their product.

We have talked about what to look for when purchasing packaged and prepared medicinal herbs. You can locate these alternatives at health food stores, dietary supplement stores, pharmacies, and even in your big chain grocery stores. While these options are a great alternative to chemicals, there is always the option of creating your own remedies at home. This option will be discussed further in Chapter Six, Growing Your Own Medicinal herbs.

If you do not have the option to garden and want to go pick some herbs, here are a few practical tips to follow.

Rule One. Identify what you are picking correctly. It is extremely easy to confuse some herbs which are indistinguishable in looks but contain very different properties for healing purposes.

Rule Two. Always pick more than a mile off the highway. There are some herbs that seem to thrive on car exhaust fumes. Plants picked next to a busy road may have up to 200 times their natural lead content.

Rule Three. If your herb of choice is growing profusely in a given area, this is a good indication that the soil is nutrient and mineral-rich which is promoting that healthy growth. Picking your herbs from areas such as these is a good choice.

Rule Four. Pick your herbs once the dew has evaporated from the leaves, around mid-morning. Many plants will develop mold after picking if there is any dampness on them.

Rule Five. Select only the best plants, avoiding the ones that display any signs of disease or damage. Drooping leaves, black spots or a discolored stem are all signs that the plant is not a healthy one.

A great advantage to using medicinal herbs as a therapy or health enhancement is that it is totally safe especially when it is administered correctly. Beware of the publicity that erroneously states that medicinal herbs can be swallowed in random amounts without any ill effects occurring. Not only is this incorrect, it is also very dangerous.

Medicinal herbs are safer than current western medications but they still must be taken with the awareness of accurate dosage. Always check with a professional what the correct dosage of medicinal herbs you should be taking. Certain plants used for benign purposes are extremely toxic and can create very harmful side effects if not taken with care. Unless you have the medical certification qualifying you to prescribe medication, do not treat anything more than a minor illness at home. Always talk to professionals about any serious health concerns. If your minor illness is not responding to your medicinal herbal remedies, you should seek professional advice. Keep in mind that if you have any doubts regarding a medicinal herb best not to take it until you can confer with an expert in herbal medicines.

Chapter 3:
External Physical Uses and the Specific Herbs

This chapter will cover six of the more common ailments that can afflict the average human. Although the frequency of these may vary with our age and our physical activity level, most of us will experience at least two of these ailments at least one time in our life.

Cuts and Bruises

Probably the number one cross-generational ailment there is. It is also one of the ones that we can be assured will go away with time.

Arnica is top of the list for its medicinal power. Used for centuries, this pretty plant can be applied topically (cream, essential oil or tincture) for treating bruises and offering some pain relief right at the source. Arnica can also be taken orally as a form of homeopathy, providing healing for physical and emotional trauma.

Comfrey is well respected in permaculture gardens as it reproduces like crazy while improving the soil at the same time. For humans, Comfrey is respected for its active ingredient, allantoin which is a compound that assists with increasing the speed of cellular growth which is extremely beneficial with the healing of cuts, bruises, and even broken bones. Comfrey is normally applied in poultice form.

Chamomile is not only a yummy cup of tea. It is also an anti-inflammatory with antibacterial properties. Wet tea bags can be applied directly to cuts for the best treatment results.

Eucalyptus is known for its consumption by koala bears and the medicinal smell of its leaves. This smell is redolent of the antiseptic properties contained in those leaves making it a good poultice for pain reduction in muscle and joint injuries or used as an ointment for small cuts. If using Eucalyptus in oil form, be sure to dilute it before applying to the affected area.

Plantain can be found all over your yard. You can easily find one if you have been bitten by a bee or spider. Chew a few leaves to get the juices flowing then apply directly to the bitten area, barring that you can find it in a tincture or salve form. Plantain is also useful for bruises and cuts.

Tea Tree oil is known for its antibacterial powers and is used as an antiseptic in hand soaps and antimicrobial in dish soaps. Originating in aboriginal Australia, this oil is very powerful when applied topically as it treats cuts and prevents the risk of infection.

Witch Hazel can be substituted for rubbing alcohol because of its astringent properties causing the damaged tissues to contract and slow or stop bleeding. This will help bruise injuries to fade faster as it speeds up the recovery time of the internal damage. Witch Hazel can be applied by soaking a cotton pad or cloth and applying directly to the area.

Yarrow has been used on battlefields to treat deep puncture wounds. It has both anti-bacterial and anti-inflammatory qualities which work on the wound to both heal and prevent scarring. Yarrow is most often found in tincture or extracts form.

Swelling, Inflammation, & Arthritis

Many of the medicinal herbs available for treating inflamed joints, whether due to injury or arthritis, are taken orally. These treatments will be covered in Chapter 4. The three mentioned here are for external use only. Apply the herb extracts directly to the afflicted area for immediate results.

Aloe Vera is most commonly known for treating small scrapes and minor burns, sunburns or heat burns. The same gel you use on your sunburn can be applied to relieve the ache in your joints.

Frankincense or Boswellia is well-known to herbal medical practitioners for the plant's anti-inflammatory properties. Derived from the Boswellia tree found in India, the gum is believed to work by blocking the substances which attack a healthy joint in autoimmune diseases like Rheumatoid Arthritis. This herb is available in a topical cream form.

Eucalyptus shows up here for the tannins found in its leaves. These tannins are useful in the reduction of swelling and pain in swollen joints. You can follow up an application of Eucalyptus with a heating pad to increase the absorption into the area. This can be found in a topical oil extract. Be sure to dilute it a little with non-medicinal oil before applying directly to the skin.

Capsaicin is the active ingredient in hot peppers. For pain relief, this ingredient works to manipulate physical pain by limiting our perception of pain, triggering endorphins to release, and offering an analgesic action. The lower concentrate creams can significantly reduce arthritic pain while those with a higher capsaicin concentration works well for peripheral nerve pain. Be careful to avoid touching the eyes or other sensitive tissue when using.

Comfrey, added here for a topical treatment for broken bones, is also known as knitbone. Used as a poultice once your bone is out of a cast or if your bone area can be accessed, comfrey leaf can be used dried or fresh, steeped in a little water and oil (to prevent the leaf from sticking to the skin) and applied directly to the skin surface and covered with gauze to hold it in place. For the best results, change the poultice every couple of hours.

Skin Health, Dry & Cracked, Burns, Eczema, Psoriasis, Insect Bites and Acne

The skin is the largest organ in our body. Many of us forget to factor in the regular maintenance of this organ when we think about our overall physical well-being. Some of the following medicinal are specific to certain conditions. Be sure to test for potential allergic reactions by applying a small amount on a part of your body 12 to 24 hours prior to use on the affected area.

Aloe Vera again appears at the top of every medicinal plant practitioners list due to the gel or fluid contained within its leaves being used for centuries as a healing agent and a topical pain-reliever. Aloe can be very effective in treating psoriasis as well as all types of burns and cracked skin.

The Calendula Flower has a history of success in treating rashes and burns and certain kinds of skin ulcers. Calendula tea can be made into a compress as well as using it topically in cream form.

Comfrey roots and leaves have shown themselves useful in the treatment of rashes. Be careful though, a topical application should not last more than three days concurrently as overuse of this plant on the broken skin can lead to toxicity in the area.

The Chamomile flower, both dried and fresh, can be used in tea form as an oral rinse to treat gingivitis and mouth lesions. Externally, chamomile in cream form works to relieve itchy lesions, sunburns, and hives. Chamomile oil mixed with oatmeal in a bath is a soothing skin treatment for eczema.

Lavender, or more specifically, Lavandula angustifolia, is widely recognized for its skin healing compounds. You can find it in cream, ointment, carrier oil, and hydrosol format for almost every skin ailment there is including psoriasis, acne, and irritated skin. You can use it as a facial steam for an anti-aging treatment.

The Marshmallow root is the more common source of this plant to be found in skin and hair formulas. It is both a source of anti-inflammatory and skin-soothing agents helpful for treating eczema, burns and moisturizing dry skin.

Rose water is known for a popular scent most typically ascribed to elderly English females. They might be on to something. Roses contain antibacterial and anti-inflammatory, making them very effective in acne-prone skin. These compounds are richly effective in anti-aging care, nourishing, hydrating, and even rejuvenating skin.

Digestion

Aids for digestion are most commonly taken orally but there is one worth mentioning as an external source of comfort.

Peppermint oil contains menthol, an active ingredient in rubs and liniments. Diluting a few drops into some massage oil (sweet almond) and rubbing over the abdominal area will have a relaxing and anti-spasmodic effect on the smooth muscles of the gastrointestinal tract.

Headaches

Headaches occur for a wide variety of reasons such as tension, dehydration, fatigue, eye strain, allergies, colds, and trauma to name a few. Many of the medicinal plant sourced remedies are taken orally but there are three methods you can try externally to ease the pain. Be sure to drink water as well as trying the following.

Peppermint Oil can stimulate a marked increase of blood flowing to the forehead while soothing muscle contractions. In combination with ethanol, Peppermint Oil can reduce your headache sensitivity. You can dilute this oil with a few drops of sweet almond or coconut oil and rub directly onto your temples, forehead, and the back of your neck.

Lavender Oil is used in this context as a mood stabilizer and very mild sedative. You can place a few drops on a cotton pad or cloth and keep close by, inhaling it every fifteen minutes or so for the best effect. You can also apply the oil in the same method Peppermint oil is used.

Apple Cider Vinegar is not traditionally known as a medicinal plant. However, it is plant sourced and used for the treatment of certain ailments. Pour two cups of the vinegar into a hot bath. This will help draw the uric acid out of your body relieving tension and headaches.

Foot Care

If you are on your feet all day there is nothing like a foot bath to freshen the feet. TI prepare a foot tea, heat one gallon of water to boiling, remove from the heat and add sixteen heaping teaspoons of fresh herb. Cover, allowing to steep for twenty minutes. Strain herbs out and soak your feet. You can also stir five drops of the herb's essential oil into warm water and soak.

Catnip will relax feet that are stressed.
Chamomile, flowers, will relieve swollen feet.
Eucalyptus leaves are deodorizing and energizing.
Ginger Root will warm chronically cold feet.
Horsetail can reduce perspiration.
Juniper is an excellent anti fungal.
Loveage works as a strong deodorizer.
Peppermint can cool feet that feel overheated while energizing tired feet.

Thyme can work as both an antifungal and a foot refresher.

Eye Care

These herbs soothe tired, red eyes while softening the delicate skin around the eye itself. Take care when using herbs around the eyes. Keep the remedy as pure as possible. Below are five herbs you can create a strong decoction with, straining it twice to ensure all little bits are removed from the liquid. Use gauze of flannel to dip in the liquid and squeeze enough so that the cloth is not dripping. Lay down to apply, leaving cloth on closed eyes for fifteen minutes.

Calendula is an extremely gentle herb, very soothing to inner eye and the skin around the outer eye. Use only the flower petals for making the decoction.

Chamomile is very effective to use when your eyes are strained from overuse.

Mallow is a very useful herb. Using as a decoction around the eyes will aid with softening the delicate skin.

Mint can assist with reducing the dark circles

under the eyes. Be careful to not get any into the eye itself when using the decoction. Carefully dab on the skin itself with a cotton ball.

Rose will soothe and calm the skin around the eyes. Be careful to use only organic roses as the ones in floral markets have been sprayed with many chemicals that will harm your skin.

For Cleaning and Refreshing your Home

Lavender is a known disinfectant, mix a little oil with water and it can be applied safely to any surface. This will leave behind a scent which will calm and ease anxiety.

Eucalyptus, Tea Tree and Lavender all possess anti-bacterial properties. You can mix a few drops of all of them in some water to create a general disinfectant which also kills mold.

Lemon juice and Mint mixed together in water will provide you with sparkling windows and a fresh smell that discourages flies from hovering close by.

Chapter 4:
Internal Use

Herbal medicine practices regularly use combinations of herbs designed to work together to increase effectiveness and reduce the side effects of the treatment. The synergy between the active ingredients is a common occurrence in these remedies creating the effect that the therapeutic result is greater than the sum of the ingredients involved. This can be noted in that many medicinal plants show up under multiple categories for healing.

Herbal medicines, when prescribed, are done so with the individual in mind. Dosage, combinations of remedies, and timelines are based on the individual's needs at the time. Be sure to inform yourself of the appropriate dose for your body size and lifestyle.

If you are choosing to treat your minor ailments without medical input, walking into the Natural medicine aisle of your local store can be daunting given the plethora of available options for internal treatments. Having some basic knowledge of what each herb is for can provide you with the tools for choosing the best option for your particular needs. All of the herbs mentioned here can be ingested in powder, capsule, pill, or dried or fresh form. Be careful to always read the recommended dosage on the label or follow the advice given to you by your health practitioner.

Liver and Digestion

Since the times of the Roman Empire, Artichoke has been used as a digestive herb and liver tonic. One of the stronger digestive herbs, it stimulates bile flow, improving digestion, and assisting the body in breaking down food and absorbing alcohol. Artichoke will help alleviate Irritable Bowel Syndrome (IBS), nausea, bloating, and constipation.

Dandelion is used for restoring potassium levels in the body acting as a natural diuretic and promoting a healthy digestive system. Coffee made from roasted Dandelion roots is widely recognized for detoxing the liver while also acting as a tonic. Tea made from dried

Dandelion leaves can assist throughout the day in the body's excretion of excess fluids.

Ginger is an amazing warming spice that is very effective for remedying many of the body's natural functions. Introduced into Europe from China during the times of the Roman Empire, this root has a revered place in traditional Chinese medicine for over 2,000 years. Consumption can alleviate motion sickness, nausea, expel gasses from the gastrointestinal tract, stomach cramps, and heartburn. The root can be purchased and grated into hot water to make a tea. You can incorporate it directly into your food or take it in capsule form for a more powerful effect.

Slippery Elm Bark was used by Native North Americans in poultices while European settlers used it to calm the digestive symptoms of people suffering from typhoid. The inner powdered bark of the elm tree is used today as a common remedy for acid dyspepsia, IBS, or any problem which may occur when you ingest a food that causes discomfort. The moisturizing property protects the stomach lining, easing diarrhea and intestinal cramps while flushing toxic wastes in the intestinal system. It can also be very helpful in healing the stomach lining when leaky gut syndrome occurs.

Milk Thistle, a flowering member of the daisy family, is used for digestion and to strengthen the liver. It has liver-protective powers which mean that it is effective for treating many liver disorders through maintaining the liver cells healthy and neutralizing the effect toxins have on this organ.

Peppermint, noted as an external digestive remedy in Chapter 3, returns here in oral form for relief from colic, a sluggish digestion, bloating, and gas. Peppermint oil is medically accepted as an effective treatment for IBS, as they can assist with easing the symptoms of cramps, bloating and spasms. Ingestion can take the form of infusions or teas and also in capsules for a more direct response to IBS symptoms.

Headaches, Muscle Tension

Butterbur has been effectively used for many years to treat tension headaches. The extract helps to reduce the intensity and frequency of headaches and is effective as a preventative for both adults and children. Butterbur contains both anti-inflammatory and antispasmodic qualities.

Feverfew contains a pain relieving biochemical called parthenopids which are known to limit the dilation of blood vessels on the head, a condition which can be the cause of severe headaches. Feverfew is very effective at minimizing the severity, frequency, and duration of headaches, migrants in particular.

Gingko Biloba is well known as a circulatory stimulant specifically for the brain. It is one of the remedies for ensuring the blood stays fluid due to an anti-platelet activity property which means it is a great source for preventing headaches caused by altitude sickness.

White Willow Bark, the active ingredient in aspirin, is an excellent choice for reducing the pain that comes with tension headaches. It is highly effective and easy on the digestive system and liver making it the preferred choice for over-the-counter choices.

Devil's Claw, from South Africa, is a plant with medicine right in its roots. The plant is very good at relieving muscle tension in the neck, shoulders, and back. It can be taken in tincture or extract form.

Chamomile has 36 flavonoids, compounds which act as an anti-inflammatory. Drinking a cup of Chamomile tea will help reduce the spasms in muscles, thus alleviating pain.

Cherry Juice is very effective at minimizing muscular stress created by physical activity. Tart cherry juice will reduce pain. The antioxidants and anti-inflammatory also assist the muscles to relax to alleviate muscular tension.

Bones & Joints

All joint ailments benefit from an increased intake of essential fatty acids. This can be done by increasing your Omega 3 intake through a variety of oils available or through the supplements listed below.

Burdock Root contains sterols, tannins, and essential fatty acids. These all add up to its reputation as an anti-inflammatory. You can chop up the fresh root and use it in stir fry or make a decoction with the dried root. This herb is also available in capsule form.

Flaxseed Oil is the best option for a vegan source of Omega-3's which are essential to fight inflammation and build a healthy immune system. Note that the body absorbs the oil form much more easily than breaking down the seeds. Never cook flax or heat.

Tumeric is also an extremely effective herb for relieving joint inflammation and an effective pain remedy. It contains at least two of the same compounds found often in prescribed anti-inflammatory. Its effectiveness is the reason why it is readily used for treating cataracts, cancer, and Alzheimer's.

Stinging Nettle is another extremely effective herb used in the treatment of arthritis and gout. Anti-inflammatory properties combined with the minerals boron, calcium, silicon, and magnesium ease pain and assist in the building of a strong bone structure. Taken in leaf tea, it can help to alleviate and decrease water retention and inflammation in addition to fostering the healthy functioning of the kidneys and adrenal glands.

Licorice works very much like the body's own corticosteroids (anti-inflammatories). It can decrease the number of free radicals at the point of injury and inhibit enzyme production, a normal part of the inflammatory reaction. Licorice will also partner with the body's own release of cortisol, a naturally occurring reaction to suppress the immune system, thereby easing pain and arthritic flare-ups. It can also work to inhibit a few of the side effects of cortisol such as adrenal fatigue and resulting anxiety. Licorice can be ingested as a tea or in pill form.

Horsetail is the plant with the highest source of silica, a compound known to improve the integral tissue of the bone. It can assist with bone repair and control calcium absorption. It is best to take this in a three-week on, one-week off cycle to prevent any strain on the kidneys.

Alfalfa leaves are an excellent source of plant-based minerals essential for bone health such as calcium, magnesium, zinc, boron, and silica. The leaf is a good source of phytoestrogens, compounds used to balance out any hormonal fluctuations which can create bone ailments.

Yarrow is used in addition to the two herbs mentioned above as it increases the circulation of blood to the injured area. This is best taken in a tincture or tea form.

Comfrey, otherwise known as knit-bone, is an herb known for its rapid bone healing properties. Taken orally as soon as the injury occurs will assist in a quick recovery.

Red Clover is known to work well for people with osteoporosis due to it being a good source of phytoestrogens and minerals. Research has shown that women taking a regular supplement of red clover isoflavones developed significantly lower rates of spinal bone loss than the subjects in the placebo group.

Heart, Blood and Circulatory System

Cayenne Pepper is a favorite among herbal medical practitioners for increasing blood circulation and as a blood cleanser. As stimulate for the circulatory system, it works by dilating the blood vessels, thus increasing blood flow throughout the body. This herb can be added to your cooking or taken in pill form.

Ginger works as a nice alternative if the cayenne pepper is a bit too strong. This gentle warming herb activates blood circulation by thinning the blood. One Japanese study found it beneficial for improving the blood flow in the intestines themselves. Drinking a few cups of ginger tea each day is a nice way to stimulate your circulation system.

Prickly Ash bark is a very effective remedy for improving poor circulation of the blood resulting in cold hands and feet. The active compounds stimulate the central nervous system improving blood flow throughout the whole body.

Hawthorn has been used for years in the

treatment of heart disease, mild congestive heart failure, and irregular heartbeats. The bioflavonoids occurring in Hawthorn assist in the dilation of blood vessels which protects them from free radicals, generally improving circulation throughout the whole body.

Garlic is one of the most versatile of the medicinal plants. Raw garlic contains high quantities of allicin, used to improve blood flow while also working as a diuretic to flush out excess fluids. Studies out of Britain have shown that garlic tablets increase whole body's blood circulation which results in a reduced risk of heart disease.

Cinnamon is one of the medicinal herbs that has a nice taste and is used to improve the level of blood sugar in the body and circulation. Chinese medicine doctors have accessed Cinnamon for centuries as a warming agent to assist with digestion and circulation.

Coumarin is the active ingredient which contains the compounds for thinning the blood.

Rosemary is known for improving circulation amongst those with muscle pain, sciatica, and neuralgia thereby easing muscle pain. The increased circulatory benefits include skin rejuvenation and are a good supplement for rheumatic ailments.

Yarrow, as mentioned previously, can dilate the capillaries and aids in the toning of the blood vessels themselves. It works by decongesting the capillaries, affecting the flow of blood and stimulating circulation in the body's peripheral areas. When combined with Lime Blossom and Hawthorn, Yarrow works to remedy high blood pressure and prevent blood clots from forming.

Pulmonary Circulatory System

Cinnamon shows up here again as several studies have demonstrated its positive cardiovascular effects. You can take the herb in your food, as a tea, or in pill form.

Eucalyptus's active compound is cineole. The many benefits attributed to this compound are as an expectorant, relief from coughing, soothing sinus passages and fighting congestion. Since Eucalyptus also contains antioxidants, it can also support the immune system during times of illness.

Lungwort is a plant which physically resembles its name and medicinal use. Since the 1600's, Lungwort's compounds have been effectively used to clear congestion, promote lung and respiratory tract health, and guard against organisms which adversely affect respiratory health.

Elecampane, although not well known, has been used by the Greeks, Romans, Chinese, and Ayurvedic practitioners for its soothing effects on the smooth tracheal muscles. The plant's roots contain inulin which soothes the bronchial passageways and pantolactone, an expectorant and anti-cough stimulant.

Lobelia, according to some practitioners, is the single most valuable ingredients in herbal remedies to date. Containing the alkaloid lobeline, Lobelia thins out mucus, thus breaking up congestion. Further, it stimulates the adrenal glands' response to release epinephrine, relaxing the airways, and creating easier breathing. It can also relax the smooth tracheal muscles, an active component in cold and cough remedies.

Osha Root is native to the Rocky Mountains, and North American indigenous cultures have used it for respiratory support for many years. The plant's roots contain camphor, making it one of the essential lung-support herbs. It will increase the circulation to the lungs, making deep breaths occur easily.

Peppermint (oil) can be used to promote free breathing and relax the smooth muscles along the respiratory tract. Peppermint has an antihistamine effect while menthol works very effectively as a decongestant. It is also beneficial for fighting organisms due to it being an antioxidant.

In addition to everything listed above in the Pulmonary Section, here are a few choices for dealing specifically with Hay Fever.

Tinospora Cordifolia is well known in India for relieving allergies, helping to alleviate itching, sneezing, and runny nose.

Timothy Grass (Phelum Pretense) has had many studies done regarding its effectiveness. The studies demonstrate that the pollen extract taken under the tongue can aid in the elimination of hay fever and grass pollen allergy symptoms. When injected, the herb can relieve the symptoms of seasonal allergies. Studies have also supported the belief that if given regularly to children for a few years, it can lower their chances of developing asthma.

Reishi Mushroom or the mushroom of immortality is a powerful herb used for centuries by both Japanese and Chinese medicinal practitioners. Research has shown it to be very effective as an antihistamine, controlling the release of histamines in the body.

Dental Care

For centuries, herbal products have been used in dentistry as antiseptics, antioxidants, antimicrobials, antifungals, antibacterial, antivirals, and analgesics. Medicinal herbs have been very effective in the control of microbial plaque (gingivitis and periodontitis) while aiding in the overall healing processes.

Take one teaspoon each of dried rosemary, peppermint, and lavender. Mix them together well and place in one cup of boiling water. Let steep for fifteen minutes, strain, and cool. It can also be used as a mouthwash for halitosis (bad breath).

Frankincense can be chewed in the form of a gum for promoting good oral health. The compounds contained within the oil-based resin are slowly released into the mouth and digestive tract and is beneficial for their antimicrobial, anti-inflammatory, and anti-tumor qualities. Frankincense in essential oil form is a very effective mouthwash. In powder form, the herb leads to a significant decrease in inflammatory conditions, one being plaque caused gingivitis.

Goldenseal is widely used for gum infection treatment. Most effective as a mouthwash, when combined with Myrrh, can be a powerful antimicrobial to be used in cases of acute gingivitis.

Echinacea Root is an American Native remedy for a toothache. The root contains high levels of inflammatory.

Lamiaceae Herbs which include rosemary, mints, lavender and sage are all powerful tools for oral and dental health. They can be used in essential oil form (very aromatic) in mouthwashes and dry powder form for brushing. The leaves of the Sage plant are excellent when used fresh and applied to suppress bleeding of the gums, gingivitis, and sores in the mouth. Peppermint leaves can be chewed fresh for improvement of the breath and to alleviate inflammation of the gums.

Prickly Ash bark is a proven method to stop toothaches or any other mouth pain. It can quicken healing after a pulled or accessed tooth as it improves circulation to the mouth.

Women's health

Women have relied on medicinal herbs for thousands of years, long been known as the practitioners of herbal medicine. The accumulated knowledge from their passing on of this knowledge has brought the practice of herbal medicine to where it is today. Herbs play a significant role in providing support to a woman as she transitions through the periods of her life.

Dandelion is one herb that humans will never be without. It is a powerful tool as a diuretic for pre-menstrual bloating and combined with Stinging Nettle, works together to purify the blood. Dandelion root can be taken in the usual variety of pill forms or taken in coffee form.

Chaste Tree Berry is one of the best for providing support to a woman during her menstrual cycle. It acts as a hormone balancer through the support of the communication between the ovaries and the brain resulting in a healthy level of estrogen and progesterone in the body. This herb should be taken in tincture form.

Red Clover has the densest source of phytoestrogens which are useful when the body's natural estrogen levels are low, for example during menopause. This is useful for other menopausal symptoms such as hot flashes, night sweats, and vaginal dryness due to drops in estrogen levels. The fresh herb can be steeped in a tea and consumed as needed.

Black Cohosh flower essence is the most commonly prescribed herb for menopause. It can be combined with Red Clover to manage symptoms in addition to lifting one's mood. This root can be taken as a tincture, tea, or in capsule form.

Holy Basil (Tulsi) assists with lowering stress hormones (cortisol). It is very calming and can help with mental clarity. This is perfect for mothers who multi-task and are under a lot of stress. Holy Basil is a delicious tea and is used in tincture and capsule form as well.

There are some medicinal herbs which should never be taken with prescription medicine. The potentially fatal health effects are not something to ignore. This warning is given repeatedly and really should be actively followed. The is not to say that if you are taking prescription medication you can not ingest any medicinal herb supplements. Rather be mindful and always research the combinations before administering.

Some potentially adverse combinations include:

St. John's Wort and antidepressants – it can raise the serotonin levels in your body too much potentially leading to seizures, pregnancies in women on oral birth control and inhibited effectiveness of anti-cancer medication.

Fenugreek, can lower the blood sugar level too much and interfere with some medications for diabetes. Also it is a dangerous combination with anticoagulants (warfarin) because Fenugreek can also delay blood clotting.

Gingko Biloba, if taken with aspirin, fish oil or ibuprofen – all blood thinners, can increase the risk of bleeding. Gingko Biloba slows the clotting action of blood and can cause bleeding to occur.

Echinacea will counter act with prednisone. The steroid decreases the immune system while Echinacea stimulates it. You will receive no benefit from either if taken at the same time.

Chapter 5:
Emotional Health

Medicinal herbs are often thought of as treatments for what physically ails us, boost our immune system, alleviate pain, fix our digestive problems and overall, support our physical wellbeing. It is well known that our physical body and our mental/emotional bodies are intertwined. What is happening in one will affect the other two. Both Chinese and Ayurvedic medicine practices support the theory that you cannot address an ailment without looking at all three areas of your life.

When using medicinal herbs to improve your emotional well being, look for ones that include hormone balancing properties and improve liver and gallbladder function. It is always best to work with an experienced herbal practitioner when taking herbs for mentally therapeutic purposes with deep roots. The following have been selected for their use to relieve anxiety, lift your mood, promote sleep and calmness, and to improve focus or clarify mental functions.

Sleep Aids

Lemon Balm, when consumed in tea form, has been traditionally used to treat insomnia and anxiety. It is more recently found to calm people with Alzheimer's disease who suffer from agitation.

Valerian is frequently combined with Lemon Balm, creating a mild but effective sedative for people who struggle with insomnia. It can also be taken on its own in tea form.

Catnip appears to have the opposite effect on humans that it has on cats, as humans only experience calming effects. These include relief from stress and anxiety, helps with migraines, and assists in the treatment of insomnia. You can mix the catnip with chamomile leaves to strengthen its relaxing power.

Anxiety and Stress

The herbs mentioned above are effective for responding to and improving anxiety and stress. Their only drawback is they are also effective sleep aids. The following listed here are also effective without creating drowsiness.

Lavender is a very popular herb used to calm the nerves. Essential oils can be used in a diffuser, scenting your surroundings in tranquility or placing the herb in a sachet to place under your pillow. Lavender scented creams can be applied and there are some who believe ingesting Lavender in pill form will help to reduce anxiety.

Passionflower, taken as a tea, can improve symptoms of anxiety, aviation, and irritability. It is also useful when experiencing opiate drug withdrawal symptoms.

Ashwagandha showed similar effects as those of the pharmaceutical drug lorazepam. A 2012 study showed that taking the plant extract in capsule form can significantly reduce cortisol levels without any serious side effects occurring.

Depression

St. John's Wort is the most prevalent herb used for the treatment of both anxiety and depression. It is well established as an effective anti-depressant, equivalent to those pharmaceutically created, with fewer side-effects.

Maca has been used in Peru for centuries to alleviate depression in men and women while increasing their libido. Some current research has found it very effective for treating symptoms of depression in women going through menopause. The plant is grouped according to its color, but the roots from all of the plants (black, red, cream) are helpful in treating this condition. Maca can be taken in tea or capsule form.

Ginseng has been a staple in the Chinese medicine chest for centuries. The modern-day root is derived from the American or the Asian plant. The qualities it possesses for reducing depression are that it boosts energy and improves mental clarity while reducing the symptoms of stress. These can help people suffering from reduced energy and motivation due to depression. Take note, people with bipolar disorder can trigger mania if taking ginseng.

Chamomile was studied in 2012 for its role in managing depression. The results showed that this herb does produce relief from symptoms of depression, perhaps through its action as a sleep aid. People have more energy and feel fewer symptoms.

Memory and Mental Clarity

Sage has long been known to sharpen the mind. There have been a number of recent studies to support this claim. Common as a Mediterranean culinary herb, Sage can improve mood and memory with a single dose and possibly protect memory and cognition functions in the brain.

Rosemary, another culinary herb from the Mediterranean, can improve cognitive function in low doses. Studies of the herb in aromatherapy use showed that the scent can aid memory and increase focus while reducing stress. Like Sage, Rosemary can also pick up your mood and protect your brain.

Gingko, taken in leaf extract form, is popular in Europe for treating a wide variety of conditions including memory loss and problems associated with concentration and confusion. Gingko is believed to work through the actions of increasing the blood supply, a reduction in blood viscosity and free radicals, and an increase in the presence of neurotransmitters.

Chapter 6:
Growing Your Own Medicinal Herbs

Gardening and herbal medicine are both age-old practice's that have been with us for thousands of years. It is interesting to note that growing the medicinal herbs produces the same benefits as taking them. Gardening can reduce stress, bolster the immune system through exercise and fresh air, keeps your mind sharp, and helps you sleep at night. The benefits of growing your own medicinal herbs are limitless, it's no wonder so many people are turning to grow their own.

The science of gardening continues to develop and with it, the art of healing with herbs. Both have gained popularity due to concerns over our current food sources and the affordability in creating one's own food and medicine source. The availability of information on plant culture, do-it-at-home recipes for herbal remedies, and new research on the multiple uses of these remedies are creating huge potential for growth for all concerned.

In the past, it was common to devote a section of the yard for growing flowers, fruit, vegetables and herbs. These plots were an integral part of the community landscape, socializing with the neighbors over the garden fence was an integral part of a family's everyday life. Frequently, sections of these gardens were wholly devoted to the growth of plants for the purpose of home remedies.

In addition to gardens being a source of the community social fabric, they also created a link between people and nature. Habitats were created to nurture the presence of insects, butterflies, birds and snakes, all necessary for plant pollination and garden health. People kept a closer watch on the weather, relying on their joints to tell them what was going to happen. By digging up a small plot in our yard, or planting pots to set on the balcony, a medicinal herb garden is an active means of staying involved with the natural world around us.

The best advice to be given is, if you are starting an herb garden for your very first time, it is always a wise choice to keep things simple. Start small, maybe five to ten plants. Make it manageable, keep it enjoyable. That way, you will enjoy gardening, finding it pleasurable and not a chore. Plants pick up on their surroundings and beautiful, healthy gardens are built by people who love being in them.

Before you start digging and planting, there are a few considerations to make. Obviously, if you are growing the plants in pots on a balcony, you will have fewer options in respect to sunlight and water source. One of the biggest mistakes you can make is to build your garden far away from a water source. It might seem appealing and back-to-the-earth appealing in the beginning, but hauling water, compost, and tools become very tiring over a season. Try to consider the distance from water to beds (or pots), access for a wheelbarrow to move compost in and weeds out, distance to the compost pile (if you are creating your own) and distance from your house. Of course, much of this will be pre-determined by your lot size but it is good to think of these points and create the most accessible herb plot you can.

The last considerations are sun and soil. How much sun will the plants receive in one day? Most medicinal herbs (not all, but most) would prefer to enjoy up to eight hours of sunshine a day, if not more. More sunshine will result in a higher concentration of oil inside the herb, creating a more potent plant. In respect to soil, is it acidic and filled with rocks? Clay? Sand? Some herbs prefer the Mediterranean conditions of a dry, less loamy soil with excellent drainage while other plants need a cool, shady environment. You can always amend the soil prior to planting, adding compost, peat moss, lime, and bone meal. Be sure to know once you have selected which plants you want to begin your garden with and research the soil and sun requirements prior to planting. This holds true if you are using containers.

One way to strategize the most effective garden is to draw it out. Whether it is round, oval or shaped like a kidney, pick something you will enjoy looking at. Select which medicinal herbs you would like to grow, look at their sun and soil requirements, and then research their growth patterns. Tall herbs will go in the back or the center of the bed or pot. Smaller herbs are placed at the front. If the plant likes to spread, make sure you leave enough room around for adequate growth. This map will help you remember what you have planted from year to year (some herbs are cut right back at the end of the growing season) and it is easy, as the garden grows, to forget what you have planted where.

One way to determine how healthy your soil is by looking for signs of earthworms. If it is a cool day and there are no worms just below the soil surface, you will need to add compost and a little sand to create better drainage for the plants. Organic compost will create healthy plants. Well-aged manure is very effective if it is at least a year old. Note that herbs will develop root rot easily as most of them prefer drier conditions so beware to not overwater in your zeal to get the plants growing.

Next, decide if you are going to start from seeds or buy seedlings. Seeds are less expensive to purchase. You can sprout them inside the house. Add a little organic soil to the cups inside an egg carton, a label of which seeds you have planted where, and place the carton on an old cookie sheet as the water will seep through the cardboard. Place these in a sunny and warm area of the house and in about three weeks, you will have sprouts. By planting more than you need, you will have choices of which plant looks the healthiest.

If you choose to buy seedlings to plant right away, make sure to pick the healthiest looking plants. Garden seedlings are often ready to plant the week you purchase them, so be careful to not leave them sitting in their pots for too long. Ask before you leave the store if the seedlings have been 'hardened off'. This phrase refers to if the plants have been outside yet. Typically, planting occurs at a time of year where the air and ground are warmer, but it is best to acclimatize your plants to the outside by leaving them outside for a few hours a day until they are used to the temperatures. You will need to do this with the seedlings you have sprouted yourself.

Plant your seedlings at least two inches apart, more if they will grow into large sprawling plants. Mint should always be planted in a large pot as it will take over your yard in a couple of years. Oregano also has a tendency to spread out and take over. It could also be easily contained in a pot. Fill the hole with a little water, gently place the seedling in the hole, and gently press the dirt done around it. Add a little more water and take a photo – your first medicinal herb garden. It will never look this sparse again.

You can choose to plant the seeds directly into the soil. If so, make sure all risk of frost is past and the soil is reasonably warm. Keep an eye out for birds and rodents, they like to watch what you are doing then follow behind and snack on the seeds.

Medicinal plants which grow very well in pots are basil, calendula, cayenne peppers, ginger, lavender, lemon balm, mint (all varieties), rosemary, sage, St. John's wort and thyme. Note that rosemary does not enjoy being transplanted. They can grow quite large so ensure that the space designated for them is large and they can live there forever. All of the others can be transplanted easily.

Some people plant herbs in concrete building blocks, this keeps the plant's roots warm and keeps them separate, also cuts down on the weeding. Another idea is to lay an old wooden ladder down on a bed and plant a different plant between each rung.

You can plant all of the above container plants in a bed along with chamomile, garlic, feverfew, echinacea, and licorice.

Chickweed, dandelion, and plantain will show up in your yard without too much effort on your part. If you are an apartment dweller, simply visit a field far away from any roads or factories, and you will locate a large assortment of these medicinal plants growing wild.

Plants requiring a fair bit more space to grow as they get big are yarrow, valerian, mullein, burdock, and marshmallow.

Most of the medicinal plants mentioned will have the desire to spread out and take over. At the end of the growing season, ensure there is adequate space around each plant for room to grow the next season. It is very important to be a bit ruthless as healthy plants are the ones with adequate access to water and sunshine. If they are competing with others in the garden, you may lose one or two quieter herbs to more dominant varieties.

Your herbs might be in a competition for garden space but you should never feel you are competing for a gardening award. Keep in mind that if you are not enjoying gardening, you will not be reaping the peripheral benefits of having a medicinal herb garden. Harvesting your own herbs for use in your home should be a gratifying experience, allowing you to continue developing your garden and the options of remedies it can provide you with.

At varying times through the summer, you will be harvesting flowers, leaves. or roots from your plants for the creation of your home remedies. What follows is a basic guide to follow for the proper harvesting techniques to ensure you have the best quality materials from which to create your recipes.

You will only need to harvest the whole plant if you are requiring the roots. Otherwise, you should always only take only small amounts from each plant until your garden is well established. Then, larger harvests can be successfully undertaken as your plants will be hardy enough to sustain a larger leaf/flower loss without destroying the plant. Newer plants will only handle smaller harvesting as they are too small to sustain a whole-scale loss of leaves or flowers.

Flowerheads are prone to damage, from insects, birds, wind, or absentminded gardeners. Try to pick flowers in the morning and dry them at the first opportunity to prevent mold from growing. Any blooms that are already starting to lose their petals are past their prime and should be avoided.

Choice leaves for picking are the ones which have a healthy appearance. Biannual plant leaves should only be selected in their second year.

When you have harvested the parts of the plant you need, leaves, flowers, and seeds, store them in small cotton bags with wire frame placed inside so the leaves are not crushed or damaged.

Never mix two herbs in the same bag. They can look entirely different in your kitchen than they can in the field.

You will now need to prepare your herbs for storage as soon as possible. This is to prevent mold and mildew from growing, whereby you will have to throw out the herbs. There are many ways to preserve medicinal plants and master herbalists will each have their own method. The simplest way to store herbs is to dry them. By removing moisture from the plant, you will trap the active compounds or useful chemicals inside the plant body. This makes the plant immune to disease, mold, and other problems. Dried herbs may be stored for anywhere from three to five years without losing any of their inherent value as medicinal plants.

There are two methods for drying herbs, inside an oven or outside in the sun on a frame. The inside method is quicker, approximately one hour inside the oven as opposed to six weeks outside on the frame.

With oven drying, you will need to place your herbs on a clean, dry tray. Place a piece of aluminum foil, shiny side down, over the tray. Tuck the foil around the tray leaving only a small gap to allow moisture to escape.

Heat the oven to 150 degrees and place the tray in the oven. Take the tray out every fifteen minutes to turn the herbs over so the moisture is being evenly drawn out of the plant. When moisture is drawn out of the plant unevenly, then burning will occur. Do not let this happen. Should the plants turn brown or black, then all potency is destroyed and the plant will be useless to you.

It is very easy to over-dry or burn the plants. If you can crumble the finished, dried plant easily in your hand without it becoming powder and most, if not all, of the original color is intact, the plant is dried perfectly.

A disadvantage to this method is that herbs will lose between one-third and-one half of their potency. When the plants are dried on a frame outside, they only lose one-quarter of their original medicinal value.

For this reason, frame drying is the preferred method by experienced herbalists though it is far more time-consuming. For this option, you will require a small wood or metal box, about three-feet square, with a glass line. Line the base of the box with aluminum foil and leave a small sheltered hole for moisture to escape. Pat dry the selected herbs for drying and place on the foil, closing the lid afterward. The herbs will require turning once a day until dry, anywhere between three to six weeks.

The box should be placed in a spot with adequate sunlight and be watertight. One herb placed in the box still slightly damp will ruin the whole batch.

How you will store your herbs is determined by the method you will be using them. Ointments require powdered forms of the plant while tinctures and teas require whole roots, leave or flowers. So, a good guide to follow is that your leaves and stems are best ground, then stored while the flowers, roots, and seeds are stored whole. Be sure everything is dried thoroughly before storage.

Grinding your herbs into a powder can be done with a mortar and pestle, slower but it does allow you to decide the quality of the powder with a great deal of accuracy. An electric grinder (such as a coffee grinder) gives better uniformity to the finished product and a very fine powder.

You have now arrived at the most important step in the process. Failing to store your herbs correctly will mean you will not be able to use them. This means that all of your time and effort has been wasted.

Choose your storage room carefully. Preferably not damp, cold, or drafty nor near the kitchen as odors from cooking have been known to seep through the most airtight of containers. Never store your herbs within reach of children, they are medicine.

Choose a glass (preferably colored to keep light out), ceramic or earthenware container that is intact and airtight. Do not use anything that will allow sunlight or moisture to seep in.

Take the time to label the container carefully, as failure doing so can have fatal consequences. You should always detail the following information on the labels:

- The date when you picked the herbs. This allows you to track its potency and renew your stocks as required.

- The name of the herb, including the Latin and the common name.

- The method of drying. Since potency is affected by this, it is essential that you know the method to determine the quantity for your remedies and dosage.

- The part of the herb you have stored in the container. Ground up herbs can pretty much all look the same, though the medicinal qualities of the plant vary with the part it is contained. It is very important to know which part you have stored for use.

You are now ready to begin applying your own medicinal herbs for health and symptom relief.

Conclusion

Thank you for making it through to the end of Herbal Medicine Guide for Beginners. Let's hope it was informative and able to provide you with all of the tools you need to achieve your goals whatever they may be.

The next step is to go out and identify some of the more common medicinal herbs growing wild around you. Check out the produce department and notice the variety of the herbs available, fresh and dried. Scan your supplement aisles and acquaint yourself with the varieties of remedies available, the variation in doses, and the range of ailments which can be treated.

Next, walk around your house. Do you have space for a small plot or a few containers? Start researching how much sun your plot would get in a day and what kind of soil you have. Take stock of your medicine cabinet and notice the contents. What do you seem to require the most of in your household? Maybe plan on planting a few herbs that would meet the most common of your household requirements, cuts, bruises, insomnia.

Take your paper and start building your medicinal herb bed map so that when the next growing season arrives, you are prepared to plant your very own ingredients for those herbal remedies.

Finally, if you found this book useful in any way, a review on Amazon is always appreciated!

This book belongs to a series of books about herbal medicine and how to use it to improve our life. For more information, visit www.db-publishing.com

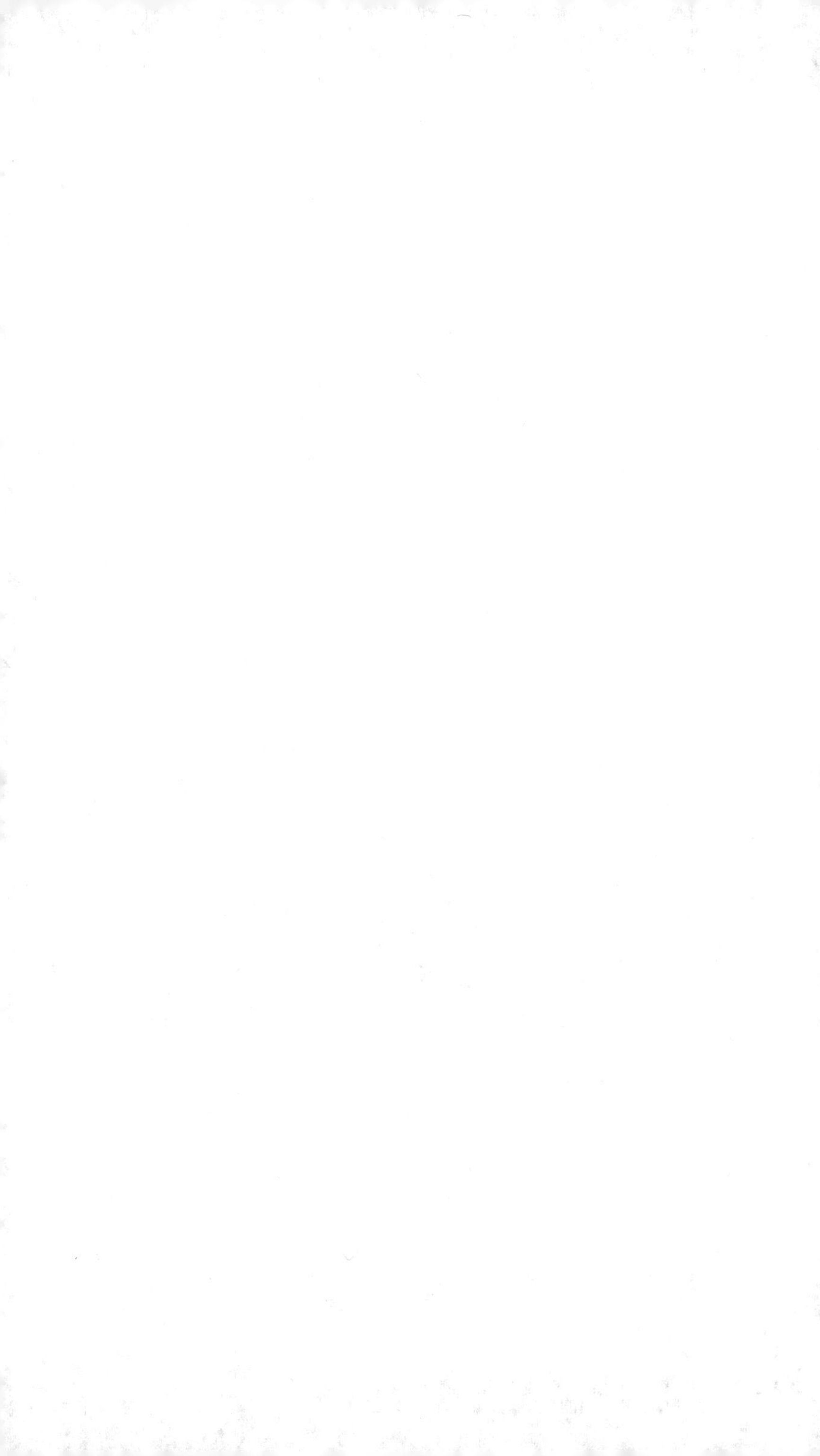